PREGNANCY AND POSTPARTUM CARE

A Comprehensive Strategy Guide For Smooth Mama Recovery & Transition

BY

DANIELLE WALLACE

Copyright Notice

TABLE OF CONTENT

LOOKING FORWARD TO THE FUTURE.......... 146

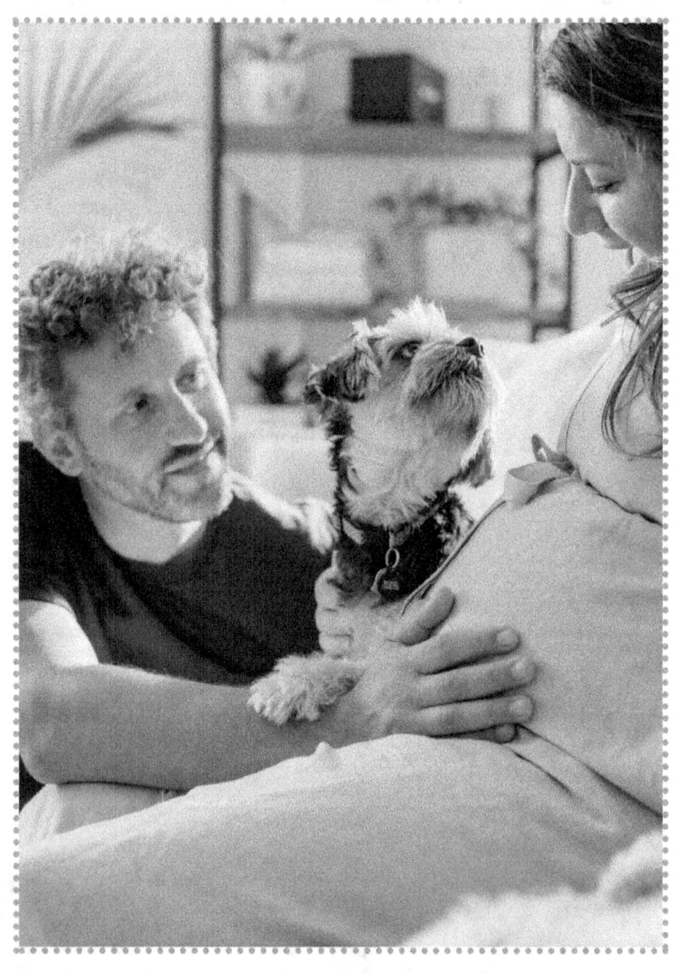

INTRODUCTION

"Pregnancy and Postpartum Care," your comprehensive guide to navigating the transformative journey of pregnancy, childbirth, and early parenthood. This ebook is crafted with the aim to empower you with knowledge, support, and practical advice as you embark on one of life's most extraordinary experiences.

Embarking on the Journey

Pregnancy marks the beginning of an incredible voyage filled with anticipation, wonder, and profound changes. From the moment of conception to the nurturing of new life within, each stage brings its own set of joys and challenges. Understanding these stages, from the early signs of pregnancy to the complexities of childbirth and beyond, is essential in preparing both physically and emotionally for the arrival of your little one.

Comprehensive Guidance

In "Pregnancy and Postpartum Care," we delve into every aspect of this journey with clarity and depth. You'll explore the physiological changes your body undergoes during pregnancy, the importance of prenatal care, and practical tips for managing common discomforts. We'll guide you through the stages of labor, help you prepare for delivery, and equip you with strategies to embrace the postpartum period with confidence.

Empowering Your Choices

Throughout this ebook, you'll find insights into making informed decisions about your health and well-being, understanding the options available to you during childbirth, and nurturing your newborn during those precious early weeks. Whether you're navigating pregnancy for the first time or seeking to enrich your experience as a parent, this ebook is designed to be your trusted companion.

Supporting Your Journey

Above all, "Pregnancy and Postpartum Care" aims to support you on your unique journey to parenthood. We recognize the importance of holistic care—physically, emotionally, and mentally—and provide resources to help you build a support network, access professional guidance, and celebrate the milestones of parenthood.

A Note of Encouragement

As you embark on this remarkable journey, remember that every experience, challenge, and moment of joy contributes to the profound tapestry of parenthood. Embrace each phase with openness and readiness, knowing that you are supported by knowledge, empowered by choice, and surrounded by a community of caregivers and loved ones.

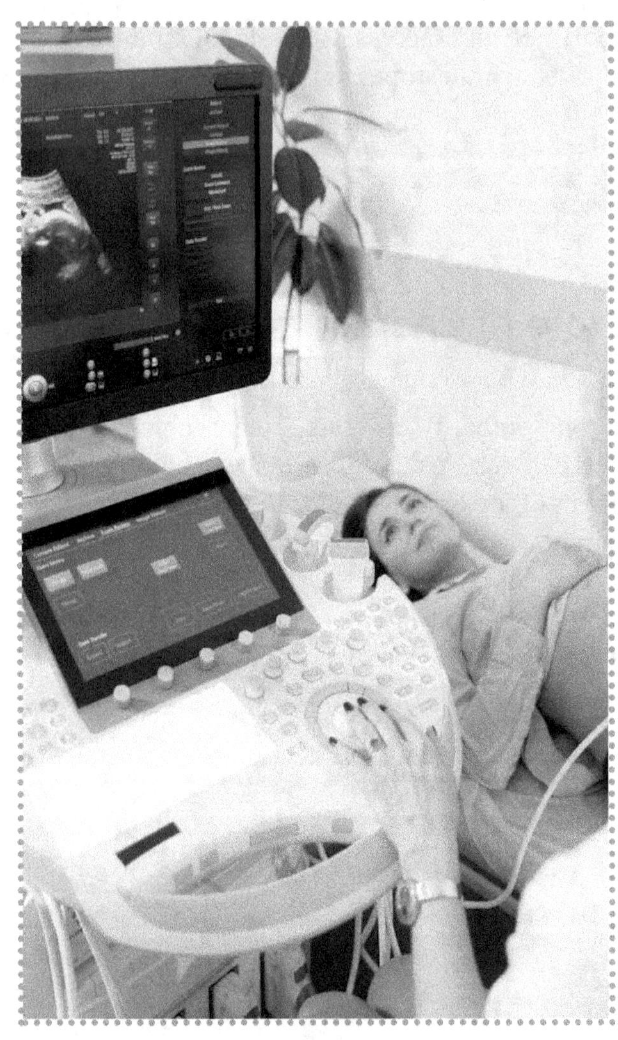

CHAPTER ONE

WELCOME TO PARENTHOOD

The Journey of Pregnancy and Postpartum

Welcome to an extraordinary chapter of your life – the journey of pregnancy and postpartum. This period is filled with profound transformations, both physically and emotionally, as you prepare to welcome a new life into the world. From the moment you discover you are pregnant, through the trimesters of development, to the intense and miraculous experience of childbirth, and finally into the postpartum phase where you and your baby begin to adjust to your new lives together, this journey is unique and deeply personal.

Pregnancy brings a series of milestones and challenges. Your body changes remarkably during the process of nurturing and growing your child.. Emotionally, you may experience a wide range of feelings, from joy and excitement to anxiety and uncertainty. Postpartum, you will face the demands of caring for a newborn while your body heals and adjusts. This time is often accompanied by a mix of elation and exhaustion, and it's crucial to recognize and address your own needs as well as your baby's.

The Purpose and Scope of the Book

This book, "Pregnancy and Postpartum Care," is designed to be a comprehensive guide to help you navigate this incredible journey with confidence and knowledge. Our goal is to provide you with reliable information and practical advice on every aspect of pregnancy and postpartum care, ensuring you feel supported and empowered throughout.

We start with an in-depth understanding of pregnancy, from the early signs and symptoms in the first trimester to the developmental milestones and physical changes in the second and third trimesters. You'll learn about the importance of prenatal care, which is essential for monitoring your health and your baby's development.

As you approach labor and delivery, we offer detailed insights into the signs of labor, the stages of childbirth, and pain management options. We also discuss the various delivery methods, potential complications, and the immediate postpartum care needed for both mother and baby.

You may discover advice on anything from nursing and basic baby care to dealing with sleep loss and postpartum mental changes in the postpartum area. We address long-term postpartum care, including physical recovery, mental health, and balancing new family dynamics.

Special considerations are covered for high-risk pregnancies, multiple pregnancies, and the unique journeys of adoption and surrogacy. Finally, we provide resources and support for building a strong support network and seeking professional help when needed.

By the end of this book, you will have a thorough understanding of the entire pregnancy and postpartum process, equipping you with the knowledge and tools to make informed decisions and care for yourself and your baby effectively. This book aims to be your trusted companion, offering support and reassurance every step of the way. Welcome to parenthood – an adventure like no other.

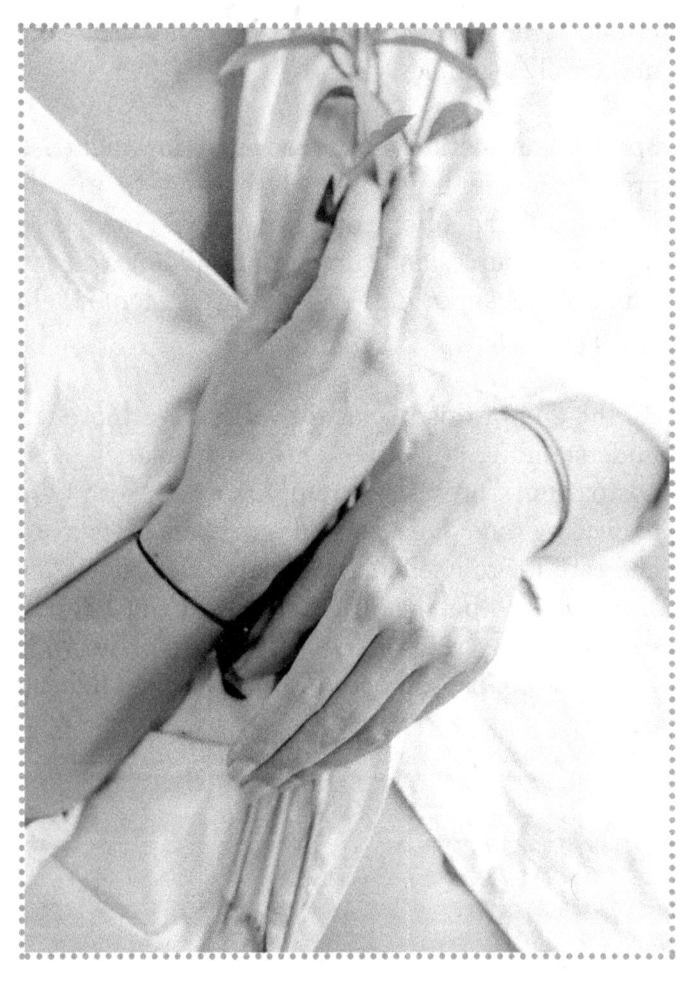

CHAPTER TWO

UNDERSTANDING PREGNANCY

Pregnancy is a remarkable and transformative journey marked by distinct stages, significant changes in the body, and the crucial role of prenatal care. In this chapter, we will explore the stages of pregnancy, the key changes your body undergoes, and the importance of regular prenatal care in ensuring a healthy and safe pregnancy.

Stages of Pregnancy

Usually, a pregnancy is broken up into three trimesters, each lasting around three months. Understanding the stages of pregnancy helps you anticipate the changes and developments that occur as your baby grows.

1. **First Trimester** (Weeks 1-12)

   ➢ **Early Development**: The first trimester begins from the first day of your last menstrual period and includes conception and early fetal development. By the end of this trimester, the baby's major organs and systems have begun to form.

> **Initial Changes**: During this period, you may experience early pregnancy symptoms such as nausea, fatigue, and breast tenderness. It is also a critical time for the baby's development, so maintaining a healthy lifestyle and attending early prenatal visits is essential.

2. **Second Trimester** (Weeks 13-26)

> **Growth and Movement**: The second trimester is often considered the most comfortable phase of pregnancy. The baby grows rapidly, and you may start to feel the baby move, usually around the 20th week.

> **Visible Changes**: You will notice your belly growing as the baby develops, and common symptoms include increased energy levels and reduced nausea. This trimester includes important screenings and diagnostic tests to monitor the baby's growth and development.

3. **Third Trimester** (Weeks 27-40)

- ➢ **Preparation for Birth**: The final trimester involves rapid growth and maturation of the baby's organs in preparation for birth. The baby gains weight quickly, and you may experience physical discomfort as your body adjusts to accommodate the growing baby.

- ➢ **Labor and Delivery**: This stage is marked by anticipation and preparation for labor and delivery. You will have frequent prenatal visits to monitor the baby's position and ensure both you and the baby are ready for birth.

Key Changes in the Body

Pregnancy brings about a multitude of changes in your body, both visible and invisible. These adjustments are required to assist your baby's growth and development.

1. Hormonal Changes

> **Human Chorionic Gonadotropin (hCG)**: This hormone is produced shortly after conception and is responsible for maintaining the pregnancy in its early stages. It is the hormone that pregnancy tests also find.

> **Progesterone and Estrogen**: These hormones increase throughout pregnancy, supporting the uterine lining, regulating the menstrual cycle, and preparing the body for breastfeeding.

2. Physical Changes

> **Weight Gain**: Gradual weight gain is expected as your body supports the growing baby, placenta, and amniotic fluid.

> **Breast Changes**: Your breasts may become larger and more tender in preparation for breastfeeding.

> **Increased Blood Volume**: Your blood volume increases to supply oxygen and nutrients to the baby, which can lead to visible veins and a rosy complexion.

➢ **Skin Changes**: You may notice changes in skin pigmentation, such as the darkening of the areolas and the appearance of a line down your abdomen known as the linea nigra.

3. Musculoskeletal Changes

➢ **Posture and Balance**: As your belly grows, your center of gravity shifts, affecting your posture and balance. This can lead to back pain and discomfort.

➢ **Joint and Ligament Changes**: The hormone relaxin loosens the joints and ligaments to prepare for childbirth, which can cause pelvic pain and instability.

Importance of Prenatal Care

Prenatal care is vital for monitoring the health and development of both you and your baby throughout pregnancy. Regular check-ups and screenings help detect and address any potential issues early on.

1. Early and Regular Visits

> **Initial Visit**: Your first prenatal visit typically occurs around 8-10 weeks of pregnancy. During this visit, your healthcare provider will confirm the pregnancy, estimate your due date, and conduct initial screenings and tests.

> **Ongoing Care**: Regular prenatal visits, usually once a month in the early stages and more frequently as the pregnancy progresses, are essential for monitoring your health and the baby's development.

2. Screenings and Tests

> **Ultrasounds**: Ultrasound scans provide visual confirmation of the baby's growth and development and can detect any anomalies or complications.

> **Blood Tests**: Routine blood tests check for conditions such as anemia, gestational diabetes, and infections that could affect your pregnancy.

➢ **Genetic Screening**: Optional genetic tests and screenings assess the risk of certain genetic disorders and congenital anomalies.

3. Health and Lifestyle Guidance

➢ **Nutrition**: Your healthcare provider will advise on a balanced diet rich in essential nutrients such as folic acid, iron, calcium, and DHA to support the baby's development.

➢ **Exercise**: Regular, moderate exercise is encouraged to maintain fitness, reduce pregnancy discomfort, and prepare for labor.

➢ **Avoiding Risks**: Prenatal care includes guidance on avoiding substances and activities that could harm the baby, such as smoking, alcohol, certain medications, and unsafe foods.

By understanding the stages of pregnancy, recognizing the key changes in your body, and adhering to recommended prenatal care, you can ensure a healthy and positive pregnancy experience. This foundational knowledge sets the stage for the more detailed information and practical advice provided in the following chapters.

PART 1- PREGNANCY

CHAPTER THREE

FIRST TRIMESTER

The first trimester marks the beginning of your pregnancy journey and is filled with significant changes and developments. This chapter will guide you through the early signs and symptoms, what to expect during your first prenatal visit, essential nutrition and lifestyle changes, and effective ways to manage morning sickness and fatigue.

Early Signs and Symptoms

The first trimester encompasses the first 12 weeks of pregnancy, starting from the first day of your last menstrual period. During this time, your body undergoes numerous changes to support the developing embryo. Here are some common early signs and symptoms of pregnancy:

1. **Missed Period**: One of the most obvious signs of pregnancy is a missed period. However, this can sometimes be accompanied by light spotting known as implantation bleeding.

2. **Nausea and Vomiting**: Often referred to as "morning sickness," nausea and vomiting can occur at any time of the day and are common during the first trimester.

3. **Fatigue**: Increased levels of the hormone progesterone can make you feel more tired than usual.

4. **Breast Changes**: Your breasts may become swollen, tender, and sensitive as they prepare for breastfeeding.

5. **Frequent Urination**: As your uterus grows and hormonal changes increase blood flow to the pelvic area, you may find yourself needing to urinate more often.

6. **Mood Swings**: Hormonal fluctuations can lead to changes in mood, making you feel more emotional or irritable.

7. **Food Cravings and Aversions**: You might experience strong cravings for certain foods or aversions to others, often due to hormonal changes.

FIRST PRENATAL VISIT:
What to Expect

Your first prenatal visit is a crucial step in ensuring a healthy pregnancy. This appointment typically occurs between the 8th and 10th week of pregnancy and involves several important components:

1. **Medical History**: Your healthcare provider will take a detailed medical history, including information about your menstrual cycle, previous pregnancies, medical conditions, medications, and lifestyle habits.

2. **Physical Exam**: A comprehensive physical exam, including checking your weight, blood pressure, and a pelvic exam, will be conducted.

3. **Confirming the Pregnancy**: An ultrasound may be performed to confirm the pregnancy, estimate the due date, and check for a heartbeat.

4. **Lab Tests**: Blood and urine samples will be taken to test for various conditions such as anemia, blood type, Rh factor, and infections. Additionally, your healthcare provider will check for immunity to certain diseases like rubella.

5. **Discussion of Symptoms**: Be prepared to discuss any symptoms you are experiencing, as well as any concerns or questions you may have.

6. **Prenatal Vitamins**: Your provider will likely recommend prenatal vitamins, especially those containing folic acid, which is crucial for preventing neural tube defects.

7. **Next Steps**: You will receive information about what to expect in the coming weeks, including scheduling future prenatal visits and any additional tests or screenings.

NUTRITION AND LIFESTYLE CHANGES

Maintaining a healthy lifestyle and proper nutrition during the first trimester is vital for your well-being and your baby's development. Here are some key points to consider:

1. **Balanced Diet**: Focus on a diet rich in fruits, vegetables, whole grains, lean proteins, and dairy. Ensure you are getting essential nutrients such as folic acid, iron, calcium, and omega-3 fatty acids.

2. **Hydration**: Drink plenty of water to stay hydrated and support increased blood volume.

3. **Avoid Harmful Substances**: Stay away from alcohol, tobacco, and recreational drugs. Limit caffeine intake to 200 mg per day (about one 12-ounce cup of coffee).

4. **Safe Food Practices**: Avoid foods that may pose a risk of foodborne illness, such as raw or undercooked meats, unpasteurized dairy products, and certain types of fish high in mercury.

5. **Prenatal Vitamins**: Continue taking prenatal vitamins as recommended by your healthcare provider.

6. **Physical Activity**: Engage in regular, moderate exercise like walking, swimming, or prenatal yoga to maintain fitness and reduce stress.

Prior to beginning a new fitness program, always get advice from your healthcare physician.

MANAGING MORNING SICKNESS AND FATIGUE

Morning sickness and fatigue are common during the first trimester, but there are ways to manage these symptoms effectively:

1. **Morning Sickness**:

   > **Small, Frequent Meals**: Eat small, frequent meals throughout the day to keep your blood sugar levels stable.

   > **Stay Hydrated**: Drink fluids between meals rather than with meals to avoid overfilling your stomach.

   > **Ginger and Peppermint**: Ginger tea, ginger candies, and peppermint can help alleviate nausea.

➢ **Avoid Triggers**: Identify and avoid foods or smells that trigger nausea.

➢ **Rest**: Rest when needed and avoid sudden movements that might worsen nausea.

2. **Fatigue**:

➢ **Rest and Sleep**: Prioritize getting adequate sleep each night and take short naps if needed during the day.

➢ **Healthy Snacks**: Keep healthy snacks on hand to maintain your energy levels throughout the day.

➢ **Gentle Exercise**: Engage in gentle exercise to boost your energy levels and improve sleep quality.

➢ **Listen to Your Body**: Recognize the cues from your body and take a break when you're feeling worn out.

Understanding the early signs and symptoms of pregnancy, knowing what to expect during your first prenatal visit, making essential nutrition and lifestyle changes, and finding effective ways to manage morning sickness and fatigue, you can navigate the first trimester with greater ease and confidence. This foundational knowledge will support you through the early stages of pregnancy, setting the stage for a healthy and positive experience as you continue your journey into the second trimester.

CHAPTER FOUR

SECOND TRIMESTER

The second trimester of pregnancy, spanning weeks 13 to 26, is often considered the most enjoyable phase. Many women experience relief from the intense symptoms of the first trimester and enjoy renewed energy levels. This chapter will cover the baby's development milestones, common physical changes and discomforts, essential prenatal tests and screenings, and the importance of exercise and maintaining energy levels during this period.

DEVELOPMENT MILESTONES FOR THE BABY

The second trimester is your baby's time for tremendous growth and development. Here are some key milestones:

1. **Weeks 13-16**:

> **Growth Spurt**: Your baby grows rapidly in length and weight. By the end of week 16, your baby is about the size of an avocado.

> **Developing Features**: Facial features become more defined. The baby's eyes and ears move to their correct positions, and the baby can make facial expressions.

> **Movements**: The baby starts to move more, though you may not feel it yet.

2. **Weeks 17-20**:

> **Quickening**: Around week 18-20, you may begin to feel your baby's movements, known as quickening.

> **Sensory Development**: The baby's senses start to develop. The brain begins to design specialized areas for smell, taste, hearing, vision, and touch.

➢ **Gender Reveal**: By week 20, the baby's gender can often be determined via ultrasound.

3. Weeks 21-24:

➢ **Significant Growth**: The baby continues to grow in size and weight. By week 24, the baby is about the size of a cantaloupe.

➢ **Organ Development**: The lungs are developing, though they won't be fully functional until later in pregnancy. The baby's skin is still translucent but will start to become more opaque.

➢ **Hearing**: The baby can hear sounds from outside the womb and may respond to familiar voices and music.

4. **Weeks 25-26:**

- ➤ **Fine-Tuning**: The baby's organs and systems are fine-tuning. The nervous system is rapidly developing, preparing for the baby to survive outside the womb.

- ➤ **Increasing Activity**: You may notice more pronounced movements and kicks as the baby becomes more active.

- ➤ **Viability**: By the end of the second trimester, the baby reaches a point of viability, meaning it has a chance of survival outside the womb with medical intervention.

COMMON PHYSICAL CHANGES AND DISCOMFORTS

As your baby grows, your body continues to change. Here are some common physical changes and discomforts during the second trimester:

1. Abdominal Growth:

> **Bump Growth**: Your baby bump becomes more noticeable as your uterus expands to accommodate the growing baby.

> **Skin Changes**: You may experience itching and stretch marks as your skin stretches.

2. Breast Changes:

> **Continued Growth**: Your breasts continue to grow and may feel fuller as they prepare for breastfeeding.

➤ **Colostrum**: Some women may begin to produce colostrum, a yellowish fluid that precedes breast milk.

3. Circulatory Changes:

➤ **Increased Blood Flow**: Increased blood volume can cause your veins to become more visible and may lead to swelling in your legs and feet (edema).

4. Common Discomforts:

➤ **Back Ache**: Back discomfort may result from the increased weight and changed center of gravity.

Maintaining good posture and using supportive pillows can help alleviate discomfort.

➤ **Leg Cramps**: You may experience leg cramps, especially at night. Stretching and staying hydrated can help reduce these cramps.

➢ **Heartburn and Indigestion**: Hormonal changes can relax the muscles of the digestive tract, leading to heartburn and indigestion. Eating smaller, more frequent meals and avoiding spicy or acidic foods can help manage these symptoms.

PRENATAL TESTS AND SCREENINGS

The second trimester includes several important prenatal tests and screenings to monitor your baby's development and detect any potential issues:

1. Ultrasound:

➢ **Anatomy Scan**: Around 18-20 weeks, a detailed ultrasound called the anatomy scan is performed to check the baby's physical development and to identify any abnormalities. The baby's gender can also be determined by this scan.

2. **Blood Tests**:

> **Quad Screen**: This blood test measures four substances in your blood to assess the risk of certain genetic conditions, such as Down syndrome, trisomy 18, and neural tube defects.

> **Glucose Screening**: Between 24-28 weeks, a glucose screening test is performed to check for gestational diabetes. You will be asked to drink a sugary solution, and your blood sugar levels will be measured.

3. **Amniocentesis**:

> **Diagnostic Test**: If indicated, an amniocentesis may be offered to diagnose certain genetic conditions. This test involves taking a small sample of amniotic fluid for analysis.

4. **Fetal Monitoring**:

> **Heart Rate Monitoring**: Your healthcare provider will regularly check the baby's heart rate using a Doppler device or

during ultrasound exams to ensure the baby's heart is functioning properly.

Importance of Exercise and Maintaining Energy Levels

Staying active and maintaining your energy levels during the second trimester is beneficial for both you and your baby. Here's why exercise and energy management are important:

1. Benefits of Exercise:

> **Improved Mood**: Exercise releases endorphins, which can help improve your mood and reduce stress and anxiety.

> **Enhanced Stamina**: Regular physical activity helps build stamina, which can be beneficial during labor and delivery.

> **Reduced Discomfort**: Exercise can help alleviate common discomforts such as back pain, constipation, and swelling.

2. Safe Exercises:

> **Walking**: A low-impact exercise that helps maintain cardiovascular health and can be done throughout pregnancy.

> **Swimming**: Easy on the joints and a great full-body workout.

> **Prenatal Yoga**: Improves flexibility, strength, and relaxation, while also preparing your body for labor.

> **Strength Training**: Light weights and resistance exercises can help maintain muscle tone and support your changing body.

3. Maintaining Energy Levels:

> **Balanced Diet**: Eating a balanced diet with a variety of nutrients helps keep your energy levels stable. Add meals high in complex carbs, protein, and iron.

➢ **Hydration**: Drink plenty of water throughout the day to stay hydrated and prevent fatigue.

➢ **Rest**: Get adequate sleep each night and take short naps if needed. When you feel exhausted, pay attention to your body and take a break.

➢ **Small, Frequent Meals**: Eating smaller, more frequent meals can help maintain steady energy levels and prevent blood sugar dips.

The second trimester is a time of significant growth and development for both you and your baby. By understanding the development milestones, being aware of common physical changes and discomforts, staying on top of essential prenatal tests and screenings, and prioritizing exercise and energy management, you can enjoy this phase of pregnancy with confidence and preparedness. This knowledge sets a solid foundation as you move forward into the third trimester, where you will begin preparing for the arrival of your baby.

CHAPTER FIVE

THIRD TRIMESTER

The third trimester, spanning weeks 27 to 40, is the final stretch of your pregnancy journey. This chapter will guide you through preparing for labor and delivery, understanding common late-pregnancy symptoms, packing your hospital bag, and making informed choices about your birth plan.

Preparing for Labor and Delivery

As you approach the end of your pregnancy, it's essential to prepare for labor and delivery. The following actions will assist you in preparing:

1. Childbirth Education Classes:

> **What to Expect**: Enroll in childbirth education classes to learn about the stages

of labor, delivery methods, and pain management options.

- ➢ **Breathing and Relaxation Techniques**: These classes often teach breathing exercises and relaxation techniques to help you manage labor pain.

2. **Hospital Tour**:

- ➢ **Familiarize Yourself**: Take a tour of the hospital or birthing center where you plan to deliver. This will help you become familiar with the facilities and policies.

- ➢ **Pre-Registration**: Many hospitals offer pre-registration to streamline the admission process when you go into labor.

3. **Birth Plan**:

- ➢ **Preferences and Choices**: Create a birth plan outlining your preferences for labor and delivery, including pain management, birthing positions, and any special requests.

➤ **Flexibility**: Remember that while a birth plan is helpful, it's essential to remain flexible as labor and delivery can be unpredictable.

4. Practice Labor Positions:

➤ **Comfort and Progress**: Practice different labor positions that can help manage pain and promote the progression of labor, such as squatting, kneeling, and using a birthing ball.

Common Late-Pregnancy Symptoms

During the third trimester, you may experience several common symptoms as your body prepares for childbirth. Here are some of the most typical late-pregnancy symptoms:

1. **Braxton Hicks Contractions**:

Practice Contractions: These are mild, irregular contractions that help prepare your uterus for labor. Although they might be painful, they are typically painless.

2. **Increased Discomfort**:

> **Back Pain**: As your baby grows, the added weight can cause back pain. Use supportive pillows and practice good posture to alleviate discomfort.

> **Pelvic Pressure**: You may feel increased pressure in your pelvis as your baby moves lower in preparation for birth.

3. **Swelling** (Edema):

> **Fluid Retention**: Swelling in your feet, ankles, and hands is common. Elevate your feet, stay hydrated, and avoid standing for long periods to reduce swelling.

4. **Frequent Urination**:

> **Bladder Pressure**: The baby's position can put pressure on your bladder, causing you to urinate more frequently.

5. **Shortness of Breath**:

> **Lung Compression**:bAs your uterus expands, it can press against your diaphragm, making it harder to breathe deeply. Practice good posture and slow, deep breathing to help.

PACKING THE HOSPITAL BAG

Packing your hospital bag in advance ensures you are ready when it's time to go to the hospital. Here's a list of essentials to include:

1. For You:

> **Comfortable Clothing**: Bring loose, comfortable clothing for labor and postpartum, including a robe, nightgown, and nursing bras.

> **Personal Care Items**: Pack toiletries, such as toothbrush, toothpaste, hairbrush, lip balm, and skincare products.

> **Entertainment**: Bring items to help pass the time, such as a book, magazine, or tablet.

> **Important Documents**: Include your ID, insurance information, and any necessary paperwork for the hospital.

2. For Your Partner:

> **Comfortable Clothing**: Pack a change of clothes and personal care items for your partner.

> **Snacks and Drinks**: Bring snacks and drinks to keep your partner energized during labor.

3. For the Baby:

> **Clothing**: Bring a few outfits, including onesies, socks, and a hat.

> **Blanket**: Pack a soft blanket to keep your baby warm.

> **Car Seat**: Ensure you have a properly installed car seat to safely bring your baby home.

BIRTH PLANS AND CHOICES FOR DELIVERY

Making informed choices about your birth plan and delivery options is crucial for a positive birthing experience. Here are some key considerations:

1. Delivery Method:

> **Vaginal Birth**: The most common method of delivery, where the baby is born through the birth canal.

> **Cesarean Section** (C-Section): A surgical procedure where the baby is delivered through an incision in the abdomen and uterus. This may be planned or arise as a need during labor.

2. Pain Management:

> **Medicated Options**: Options include epidurals, spinal blocks, and IV pain medications.

> **Non-Medicated Options**: Options Techniques such as breathing exercises,

hydrotherapy, massage, and using a birthing ball can help manage pain naturally.

3. Labor Support:

> **Birth Partner**: Your birth partner can provide emotional support, help with comfort measures, and advocate for your wishes.

> **Doula**: Consider hiring a doula, a trained professional who provides continuous physical, emotional, and informational support during labor and delivery.

4. Special Requests:

> **Labor Preferences**: Include any preferences for labor positions, use of birthing aids (such as a birthing ball), and who you want present during delivery.

> **Post-Birth Care**: Specify your wishes for immediate skin-to-skin contact, delayed cord clamping, and breastfeeding initiation.

By preparing for labor and delivery, understanding common late-pregnancy symptoms, packing your hospital bag in advance, and making informed choices about your birth plan and delivery options, you can approach the final weeks of pregnancy with confidence and readiness. This preparation sets the stage for a smoother labor and delivery experience, helping you feel empowered and supported as you welcome your baby into the world.

PART 2- LABOR AND DELIVERY

CHAPTER SIX

PREPARING FOR BIRTH

As you approach the end of your pregnancy, it's important to prepare for the birth of your baby. Understanding the signs of labor, the stages of labor, pain management options, and the role of the birth partner can help you feel more confident and ready for the big day. This chapter will cover these essential topics to ensure you are well-prepared for the birth of your child.

Signs of Labor

Recognizing the signs of labor is crucial so you know when it's time to head to the hospital or birthing center. The main indicators to watch out for are as follows:

1. **Regular Contractions**:
   - **Frequency and Intensity**: Labor contractions occur at regular intervals and

gradually increase in frequency, duration, and intensity. Unlike Braxton Hicks contractions, they do not go away with rest or hydration.

➢ **Timing**: Track the timing of your contractions. True labor contractions typically occur every 5-10 minutes and last about 30-70 seconds.

2. **Water Breaking**:

➢ **Amniotic Fluid**: Your water breaking refers to the rupture of the amniotic sac, which releases amniotic fluid. This can be a gush of fluid or a slow trickle. Contact your healthcare provider immediately if this happens.

3. **Mucus Plug**:

➢ **Cervical Changes**: The mucus plug that seals your cervix during pregnancy may be expelled as your cervix begins to dilate. This can appear as a thick discharge that may be tinged with blood, known as the "bloody show."

4. Back Pain:

> **Lower Back Pain**: Persistent lower back pain, often radiating to the abdomen, can be a sign of labor, especially if it is accompanied by other labor symptoms.

5. Pelvic Pressure:

Increased Pressure: You may feel increased pressure in your pelvis and rectum as the baby moves lower into the birth canal.

Stages of Labor

Labor is divided into three main stages, each with distinct phases. Understanding these stages can help you know what to expect and how to manage each phase.

1. First Stage:

➤ **Early Labor**: The cervix begins to dilate and efface (thin out). Contractions are mild and irregular but become more consistent over time. This phase can last several hours to days.

➤ **Active Labor**: The cervix dilates from 4 to 7 centimeters. The contractions intensify, become more frequent, and become closer together. This phase typically lasts 4-8 hours.

➤ **Transition**: There is an 8 to 10 centimeter dilation of the cervix. Contractions are intense and very close together. This is the shortest but most intense phase, lasting 30 minutes to 2 hours.

2. Second Stage:

➤ **Pushing and Delivery**: Once the cervix is fully dilated, you will start pushing to help your baby move through the birth canal. This stage can last from a few minutes to several hours, depending on whether you are a first-time mother and other factors.

3. Third Stage:

> **Delivery of the Placenta**: After your baby is born, you will continue to have mild contractions to help deliver the placenta. This stage usually lasts 5-30 minutes.

PAIN MANAGEMENT OPTIONS

Managing pain during labor is a personal choice and there are various options available. Here are some common pain management methods:

1. Non-Medicated Options:

> **Breathing and Relaxation Techniques**: Focused breathing and relaxation techniques can help manage pain and reduce anxiety.

> **Position Changes**: Moving around and trying different positions can help relieve discomfort and promote labor progression.

> **Hydrotherapy**: Soaking in a warm bath or using a shower can help soothe labor pain.

> **Massage and Acupressure**: Gentle massage and applying pressure to specific points can help alleviate pain.

2. Medicated Options:

> **Epidural**: An epidural is a regional anesthesia that provides significant pain relief from the waist down. It is administered through a catheter placed in the lower back.

> **Spinal Block**: Similar to an epidural, a spinal block is a one-time injection that provides rapid pain relief for a shorter duration.

> **IV Pain Medications**: Intravenous pain medications can help take the edge off contractions but may cause drowsiness.

3. Alternative Methods:

> **Nitrous Oxide**: Also known as laughing gas, nitrous oxide can be inhaled through a mask to provide pain relief and relaxation.

> **TENS Machine**: A TENS (transcutaneous electrical nerve stimulation) machine delivers small electrical impulses to help reduce pain.

THE ROLE OF THE BIRTH PARTNER

The birth partner plays a vital role in providing support and encouragement during labor and delivery. Here are some ways the birth partner can help:

1. Emotional Support:

> **Encouragement**: Offer words of encouragement and reassurance to help boost the mother's confidence and morale.

> **Presence**: Simply being present and attentive can provide a sense of comfort and security.

2. Physical Support:

> **Comfort Measures**: Assist with comfort measures such as massage, applying warm or cold packs, and helping the mother change positions.

> **Hydration and Snacks**: Ensure the mother stays hydrated and has access to light snacks if allowed.

3. Advocacy:

> **Communication**: Act as a liaison between the mother and healthcare providers, helping to communicate her wishes and preferences.

> **Birth Plan**: Be familiar with the birth plan and help ensure that the mother's choices are respected.

4. **Practical Support**:

> ➤ **Logistics**: Handle practical tasks such as timing contractions, tracking progress, and managing hospital paperwork.

> ➤ **Preparation**: Help pack the hospital bag, arrange transportation, and ensure that everything is ready for the big day.

With understanding the signs of labor, the stages of labor, pain management options, and the crucial role of the birth partner, you can approach the birth of your baby with confidence and readiness. This knowledge will help you navigate the birthing process more smoothly, ensuring a positive and empowering experience as you welcome your new baby into the world.

CHAPTER SEVEN

THE BIRTHING PROCESS

The birthing process is the culmination of your pregnancy journey, bringing your baby into the world. Understanding the different methods of delivery, potential complications, and immediate postpartum care is essential for a smooth and informed birth experience. This chapter will cover vaginal delivery, Cesarean section, complications during labor and delivery, and immediate postpartum care for both mother and baby.

VAGINAL DELIVERY

Vaginal delivery is the most common method of childbirth, where the baby is born through the birth canal. Here's what to expect during a vaginal delivery:

1. **Stages of Vaginal Delivery**:

   ➤ **Labor**: The process begins with labor, which is divided into three stages: early labor, active labor, and transition. Contractions help to dilate and efface the cervix.

> **Pushing and Delivery**: Once the cervix is fully dilated, the mother begins to push during contractions to help the baby move through the birth canal.

> **Delivery of the Placenta**: After the baby is born, contractions continue to help deliver the placenta, the organ that provided nourishment to the baby during pregnancy.

2. Assistance During Vaginal Delivery:

> **Episiotomy**: In some cases, a small cut may be made in the perineum to widen the vaginal opening and facilitate delivery.

> **Forceps or Vacuum Extraction**: If necessary, these tools may be used to assist in guiding the baby out of the birth canal.

3. **Recovery**:

> ➤ **Immediate Recovery**: After delivery, the mother will be monitored for bleeding and any complications. Pain relief and stitching (if needed) will be provided.

> ➤ **Postpartum Recovery**: Vaginal delivery typically involves a shorter recovery period compared to a Cesarean section. Most women can start moving around within a few hours and can go home after a day or two.

CESAREAN SECTION: When and Why

A Cesarean section (C-section) is a surgical procedure used to deliver a baby through incisions made in the abdomen and uterus. Here are the key aspects:

1. **When a C-Section is Necessary**:

> **Medical Reasons**: A C-section may be planned or performed in emergencies for various medical reasons, such as fetal distress, placenta previa, breech presentation, or health conditions of the mother.

> **Elective C-Section**: Some women may choose an elective C-section for personal or medical reasons.

2. **Procedure**:

> **Preparation**: The mother is typically given regional anesthesia, such as an epidural or spinal block, to numb the lower half of the body.

> **Surgery**: The surgeon makes an incision in the lower abdomen and another in the uterus. These incisions are subsequently used to deliver the baby.

➢ **Closing Incisions**: After the baby is delivered, the incisions are closed with sutures.

3. **Recovery**:

➢ **Hospital Stay**: Recovery from a C-section usually involves a longer hospital stay (typically 3-4 days) compared to vaginal delivery.

➢ **Postoperative Care**: The mother will need to rest and avoid strenuous activities for several weeks. Pain management and wound care are important aspects of recovery.

COMPLICATIONS DURING LABOR AND DELIVERY

While many births proceed without issues, complications can arise. Here are some common complications and how they are managed:

1. **Fetal Distress**:
> - **Signs**: Abnormal heart rate patterns in the baby can indicate distress.

> - **Management**: Immediate interventions may include changing the mother's position, administering oxygen, or performing a C-section.

2. **Prolonged Labor**:

> - **Signs**: Labor lasting more than 20 hours for first-time mothers or more than 14 hours for subsequent births.

> - **Management**: Interventions may include medication to stimulate contractions, using forceps or a vacuum, or performing a C-section.

3. **Umbilical Cord Issues**:

> **Types**: The cord can become wrapped around the baby's neck (nuchal cord) or compressed.

> **Management**: Careful monitoring and prompt interventions, such as changing the mother's position or performing a C-section, may be necessary.

4. **Excessive Bleeding**:

> **Postpartum Hemorrhage**: Significant blood loss after delivery can be life-threatening.

> **Management**: Medications, uterine massage, and, in severe cases, surgery may be required to control bleeding.

QUICK POSTPARTUM CARE FOR THE MOTHER AND CHILD

The first few hours after birth are critical for both mother and baby. Here's what to expect:

1. **For the Mother**:

> **Monitoring**: Vital signs, uterine contractions, and bleeding are closely monitored.

> **Pain Relief**: Pain relief options are provided as needed.

> **Bonding Time**: Skin-to-skin contact and breastfeeding initiation are encouraged.

2. **For the Baby**:

> **Apgar Score**: The baby's health is assessed using the Apgar score, which

evaluates heart rate, respiration, muscle
tone, reflex response, and color.

> **Initial Care**: The baby may receive a
vitamin K injection, eye ointment, and the
first bath.

> **Feeding**: Breastfeeding is encouraged
within the first hour of birth to promote
bonding and milk production.

3. Breastfeeding Support:

> **Latching**: Nurses and lactation
consultants can assist with latching and
positioning for breastfeeding.

> **Education**: Mothers are provided with
information on breastfeeding techniques
and newborn care.

4. Emotional Support:

> **Postpartum Emotions**: It's normal to
experience a range of emotions after birth.
It is essential to have support from friends,
family, and medical professionals.

> **Postpartum Depression**: Be aware of the signs of postpartum depression and seek help if needed.

With understanding the birthing process, including vaginal delivery, Cesarean sections, potential complications, and immediate postpartum care, you can approach childbirth with greater confidence and preparedness. This knowledge will help you make informed decisions and feel more empowered as you welcome your baby into the world.

PART 3- POSTPARTUM CARE

CHAPTER EIGHT

THE FIRST FEW DAYS

The first few days after your baby is born are a time of significant adjustment and learning for new parents. This chapter will guide you through what to expect during your hospital stay, the choice between breastfeeding and formula feeding, the basics of newborn care, and understanding the emotional changes that may occur, including the baby blues.

HOSPITAL STAY AND WHAT TO EXPECT

Your hospital stay after delivery is a critical period for both you and your baby. Here's what you can anticipate:

1. **Initial Assessments**:

> **For the Mother**: After delivery, you'll be monitored for vital signs, uterine contraction, and bleeding. Pain management and wound care (if you've had a C-section) are also provided.

> **For the Baby**: Your baby will undergo initial assessments, including the Apgar score, and receive necessary interventions such as vitamin K injection and eye ointment.

2. **Rooming-In**:

> **Bonding Time**: Many hospitals encourage rooming-in, where your baby stays in your room to promote bonding and facilitate breastfeeding.

3. **Breastfeeding Support**:

> **Lactation Consultants**: Specialists are available to assist with breastfeeding, ensuring a good latch and providing guidance on feeding techniques.

4. **Education and Support**:

> **Newborn Care**: Nurses will demonstrate how to care for your newborn, including diapering, swaddling, and bathing.

> **Parental Support**: You will receive information and support regarding postpartum recovery, baby care, and feeding.

5. **Discharge Planning**:

> **Health Checks**: Before discharge, both you and your baby will have final health checks to ensure you're both ready to go home.

> **Follow-Up Appointments**: You'll be scheduled for follow-up appointments with your healthcare provider and your baby's pediatrician.

BREAST FEEDING VS. FORMULA FEEDING

Choosing between breastfeeding and formula feeding is a personal decision influenced by various factors. Here's an overview of both options:

1. **Breastfeeding**:

- ➤ **Benefits for Baby**: Breast milk provides optimal nutrition, strengthens the immune system, and promotes healthy growth and development.

- ➤ **Benefits for Mother**: Breastfeeding helps the uterus contract, reduces postpartum bleeding, and lowers the risk of certain cancers.

- ➤ **Challenges**: Some mothers may experience difficulties such as latching issues, nipple pain, or low milk supply. Lactation consultants can provide vital support.

2. **Formula Feeding**:

> ➤ **Benefits**: Formula feeding provides flexibility, allowing other caregivers to feed the baby. It also ensures that the baby receives all necessary nutrients.

> ➤ **Considerations**: Formula feeding requires preparation and sterilization of bottles and nipples. It's also important to choose the right formula type for your baby's needs.

3. **Combination Feeding**:

> ➤ **Flexibility**: Some parents choose to combine breastfeeding and formula feeding, offering the benefits of both methods and providing more flexibility.

NEWBORN CARE BASICS

Caring for a newborn involves learning new skills and routines. Here are the basics:

1. **Feeding**:

➢ **Recurrence**: Usually, newborns nurse every two to three hours. Watch for hunger cues such as rooting, sucking on hands, and fussiness.

➢ **Techniques**: Ensure proper latch if breastfeeding and follow safe formula preparation guidelines if formula feeding.

2. **Diapering**:

➢ **Frequency**: Expect to change diapers frequently, as newborns may have several wet and soiled diapers a day.

➢ **Hygiene**: Keep the diaper area clean and dry to prevent diaper rash.

3. **Sleeping**:

➢ **Sleep Patterns**: Newborns sleep a lot but wake frequently for feedings. Lay your infant on their back in a bassinet or cot to provide a secure sleeping environment.

4. **Bathing**:

- ➤ **Sponge Baths**: Until the umbilical cord stump falls off, give your baby sponge baths. Once it's healed, you can transition to regular baths.

- ➤ **Temperature**: Ensure the water is warm but not hot. Use a mild baby soap and be gentle.

5. **Comforting**:

- ➤ **Soothing Techniques**: Swaddling, rocking, and using white noise can help soothe a fussy baby.

EMOTIONAL CHANGES AND BABY BLUES

Adjusting to parenthood involves emotional changes for both parents. Understanding these changes and knowing when to seek help is important:

1. **Baby Blues**:

> - **Common Experience**: Many new mothers experience the baby blues, characterized by mood swings, crying spells, anxiety, and difficulty sleeping. These feelings typically peak a few days after birth and resolve within two weeks.

> - **Support**: Rest, support from family and friends, and self-care can help manage the baby blues.

2. **Postpartum Depression**:

> - **Signs and Symptoms**: Postpartum depression, in contrast to the baby blues, is more severe and chronic. Symptoms include extreme mood fluctuations, enduring melancholy, and trouble connecting with the infant.

> - **Seeking Help**: If you suspect you have postpartum depression, seek help from your healthcare provider. Counseling, support groups, and medication can be effective treatments.

3. **Emotional Support for Partners**:

> ➤ **Adjusting to Parenthood**: Partners also experience emotional changes and need support. Communication, shared responsibilities, and support groups can help both parents adjust.

4. **Bonding with the Baby**:

> ➤ **Attachment**: Building a strong emotional bond with your baby is crucial for their development. Skin-to-skin contact, eye contact, and responsive caregiving foster a secure attachment.

With understanding what to expect during your hospital stay, making informed feeding choices, learning the basics of newborn care, and being aware of the emotional changes that may occur, you can navigate the first few days with confidence and ease. These early days are a precious time for bonding and adjusting to your new role as a parent.

CHAPTER NINE

THE FIRST SIX WEEKS

The first six weeks after childbirth, often referred to as the postpartum period, is a time of adjustment, recovery, and learning as you settle into life with your newborn. This chapter will focus on key aspects such as physical recovery for the mother, adjusting to life with a newborn, postpartum checkups, and coping with sleep deprivation.

PHYSICAL RECOVERY FOR THE MOTHER

Recovering from childbirth is a gradual process that varies for each woman. What to anticipate in the first six weeks is as follows:

1. **Healing After Vaginal Birth**:

- ➢ **Perineal Care**: If you had a vaginal birth and an episiotomy or tear, keep the area clean and use pain relief measures as recommended by your healthcare provider.

- ➢ **Pelvic Floor Exercises**: Begin doing gentle pelvic floor exercises, such as Kegels, to promote healing and strengthen pelvic muscles.

2. **Recovery After Cesarean Section**:

- ➢ **Care for Incisions**: Maintain a dry and clean incision site. If your healthcare practitioner advises against heavy lifting or intense activity, follow their advice.

- ➢ **Mobility**: Gradually increase mobility and walking to aid in recovery.

3. **Managing Pain and Discomfort**:

- ➢ **Pain Relief**: Take pain medications as prescribed or recommended by your healthcare provider to manage discomfort.

➢ **Rest**: Adequate rest and sleep are crucial for healing. Accept help from family and friends to allow yourself time to recover.

4. **Postpartum Bleeding** (Lochia):

➢ **Duration**: Expect vaginal bleeding (lochia) for up to six weeks after childbirth. Instead of using tampons, use sanitary pads to prevent infection.

ADJUSTING TO LIFE WITH A NEWBORN

Adapting to life with a newborn can be both rewarding and challenging. Here are some tips for a smoother adjustment:

1. **Establishing Routines**:

➢ **Feeding Schedule**: Whether breastfeeding or formula feeding, establish a feeding schedule that works for both you and your baby's needs.

> **Sleep Patterns**: Newborns wake frequently to feed. Rest when your baby sleeps to manage sleep deprivation.

2. **Bonding and Interaction**:

> **Skin-to-Skin Contact**: Promote bonding through skin-to-skin contact during feeding and cuddle times.

> **Talking and Singing**: Babies respond to your voice. Talk, sing, and make eye contact with your baby to foster communication.

3. **Engaging Support Networks**:

> **Family and Friends**: Accept help and support from loved ones. Share caregiving responsibilities to lighten your load.

4. **Self-Care**:

> **Prioritize Self-Care**: Take short breaks to rest, shower, and eat nutritiously. Self-care is essential for your well-being and ability to care for your baby.

POSTPARTUM CHECKUPS

Regular postpartum checkups are important for monitoring your health and recovery. Here's what to expect:

1. Timing of Checkups:

- **First Checkup**: Schedule a postpartum checkup with your healthcare provider within the first 6 weeks after childbirth.

- **Subsequent Checkups**: Additional follow-up appointments may be scheduled to monitor ongoing recovery and address any concerns.

2. Physical Assessment:

- **Pelvic Exam**: Your healthcare provider will perform a pelvic exam to check the healing of any tears or incisions.

- **Blood Pressure and Weight**: Vital signs will be monitored to ensure they are within normal ranges.

3. **Emotional Well-Being**:

> **Mental Health Screening**: Your healthcare provider may inquire about your emotional well-being, including signs of postpartum depression or anxiety.

4. **Family Planning**: Discuss contraception options if you wish to delay or prevent future pregnancies.

COPING WITH SLEEP DEPRIVATION

Sleep deprivation is common for new parents, but there are strategies to manage it:

1. Sleep When Your Baby Sleeps:

> **Nap**: Take short naps during the day to catch up on sleep.

> **Nighttime Routine**: Establish a calming bedtime routine for your baby to promote longer stretches of sleep at night.

2. Share Responsibilities:

> **Partner Support**: Share nighttime feedings and diaper changes with your partner to divide caregiving responsibilities.

> **Accept Help**: Allow friends and family to help during the day so you can rest.

3. Create a Restful Environment:

> **Sleep Environment**: Create a peaceful, dark, and comfy sleeping environment in your bedroom.

> **Limit Stimulants**: Avoid caffeine and electronic devices before bedtime to promote better sleep.

4. Seek Support:

> **Support Groups**: Join parenting groups or online forums to connect with other parents experiencing similar challenges.

> **Professional Help**: If sleep deprivation affects your mood or functioning, discuss strategies with your healthcare provider.

NOTE: focusing on physical recovery, adjusting to life with your newborn, attending postpartum checkups, and managing sleep deprivation, you can navigate the first six weeks with greater confidence and resilience. Remember to prioritize self-care and seek support when needed as you embrace your new role as a parent.

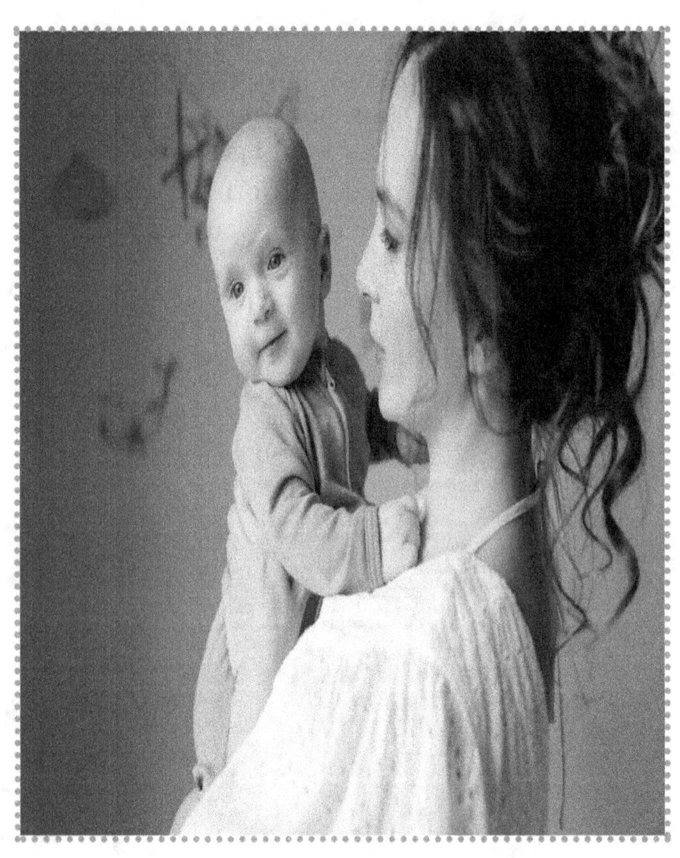

CHAPTER TEN

LONG-TERM POSTPARTUM CARE

Long-term postpartum care focuses on supporting mothers beyond the initial recovery phase, addressing mental health, physical well-being, relationships, and returning to work. This chapter will delve into managing postpartum depression and anxiety, nutrition and exercise for recovery, relationship dynamics and intimacy, and finding balance when returning to work.

Managing Postpartum Depression and Anxiety

1. **Recognizing Symptoms**:

> **Postpartum Depression**: Symptoms may include persistent sadness, irritability, loss of interest in activities, changes in

appetite, and difficulty bonding with the baby.

> **Postpartum Anxiety**: Symptoms may involve excessive worry, racing thoughts, restlessness, and physical symptoms like heart palpitations.

2. **Seeking Support**:

> **Professional Help**: Consult with a healthcare provider or therapist experienced in postpartum mood disorders.

> **Support Groups**: Join support groups or talk to other mothers who have experienced similar feelings.

3. **Treatment Options**:

> **Therapy**: Cognitive-behavioral therapy (CBT) or counseling can help manage symptoms.

> **Medication**: Antidepressants or anti-anxiety medications may be prescribed in severe cases.

4. **Self-Care Strategies**:

> **Prioritizing Self-Care**: Ensure adequate rest, nutrition, and time for relaxation.

> **Exercise**: Physical activity can alleviate symptoms of depression and anxiety.

NUTRITION AND EXERCISE FOR RECOVERY

1. Nutrition Tips:

> **Balanced Diet**: Eat a variety of fruits, vegetables, lean proteins, and whole grains to support energy levels and overall health.

> **Hydration**: Drink plenty of water, especially if breastfeeding.

2. Exercise Recommendations:

> **Postpartum Exercises**: Start with gentle exercises like walking, pelvic floor exercises, and yoga. Increase the intensity

gradually as directed by your healthcare practitioner.

> **Benefits**: Exercise promotes physical recovery, boosts mood, and helps manage stress.

3. Nutritional Considerations for Breastfeeding:

> **Caloric Intake**: Increase calorie intake if breastfeeding to support milk production.

> **Healthy Choices**: Opt for nutrient-dense foods that provide essential vitamins and minerals.

RELATIONSHIP DYNAMICS AND INTIMACY

1. Communication and Support:

> **Open Communication**: Discuss feelings, concerns, and adjustments with your partner.

> **Shared Responsibilities**: Collaborate on caregiving tasks to support each other.

2. Maintaining Intimacy:

> **Physical Connection**: Find moments for physical affection, even amidst the demands of parenting.

> **Emotional Connection**: Share experiences, listen actively, and prioritize quality time together.

3. Navigating Changes:

> **Adjusting Expectations**: Recognize that intimacy may change after childbirth. Be patient and explore new ways to connect emotionally and physically.

Returning to Work and Finding Balance

1. Planning Ahead:

> **Transition Plan**: Discuss options for maternity leave, flexible work schedules, or childcare arrangements with your employer.

> **Financial Planning**: Evaluate budgeting and childcare costs to prepare for the return to work.

2. Emotional Preparation:

> **Mixed Emotions**: Expect feelings of excitement and anxiety about returning to work while leaving your baby.

> **Support Network**: Lean on family, friends, and colleagues for emotional support during this transition.

3. **Balancing Work and Parenthood**:

- ➤ **Time Management**: Develop routines that prioritize both work responsibilities and family time.

- ➤ **Self-Care**: Maintain self-care practices to manage stress and prevent burnout.

4. **Breastfeeding Support at Work**:

- ➤ **Pumping**: Arrange for a private space and schedule breaks for pumping breast milk at work.

- ➤ **Legal Rights**: Understand your rights under workplace breastfeeding laws to advocate for your needs.

NOTE: focusing on managing postpartum mental health, maintaining a healthy lifestyle through nutrition and exercise, nurturing relationships, and navigating the return to work, mothers can promote long-term well-being and balance as they continue their journey through parenthood. Each aspect contributes to a holistic approach to postpartum care, supporting both physical and emotional health.

PART 4 - SPECIAL CONSIDERATION

CHAPTER ELEVEN

HIGH-RISK PREGNANCIES

High-risk pregnancies require special attention and care to ensure the health and safety of both the mother and the baby. This chapter focuses on identifying and managing high-risk factors, specialized prenatal care, and preparing for potential complications.

Identifying and Managing High-Risk Factors

A high-risk pregnancy is one that involves potential complications that could affect the mother, the baby, or both. Identifying and managing these factors early can help mitigate risks and improve outcomes.

1. **Advanced Maternal Age**:

> **Risk Factors**: Women over 35 are at higher risk for gestational diabetes,

hypertension, and chromosomal abnormalities.

> **Management**: Close monitoring of maternal and fetal health, including more frequent prenatal visits and specialized screenings.

2. **Medical Conditions**:

> **Pre-existing Conditions**: Conditions such as diabetes, hypertension, thyroid disorders, and autoimmune diseases can complicate pregnancy.

> **Management**: Collaborative care between obstetricians and specialists to optimize management of these conditions during pregnancy.

3. **Previous Pregnancy Complications**:

> **History of Preterm Birth**: Women who have previously delivered prematurely are at increased risk of recurrence.

> **Management**: Proactive measures such as cervical length monitoring and

progesterone supplementation to reduce the risk of preterm labor.

4. **Multiple Pregnancies**:

> **Twins, Triplets, or More**: Carrying multiples increases the risk of complications such as preterm birth, preeclampsia, and fetal growth restriction.

> **Management**: Specialized prenatal care with frequent ultrasound monitoring to assess growth and development of each baby.

5. **Genetic Factors**:

> **Family History**: Genetic disorders or chromosomal abnormalities in the family history may necessitate genetic counseling and testing.

> **Management**: Early detection through prenatal testing and counseling to provide parents with information and options.

Specialized Prenatal Care

High-risk pregnancies require specialized prenatal care to monitor and manage potential complications effectively.

1. Comprehensive Assessment:

> **Initial Evaluation**: A thorough medical history and physical examination to identify risk factors and establish a care plan.

> **Diagnostic Testing**: Additional tests such as genetic screening, fetal ultrasound, and fetal monitoring to assess fetal well-being.

2. Consultation with Specialists:

> **Multidisciplinary Approach**: Collaboration between obstetricians, maternal-fetal medicine specialists, neonatologists, and other healthcare providers.

> **Individualized Care**: Tailoring care plans to address specific risks and optimize outcomes for both the mother and the baby.

3. **Monitoring and Surveillance**:
   - ➢ **Regular Prenatal Visits**: More frequent visits to monitor maternal health indicators (blood pressure, glucose levels) and fetal growth.

   - ➢ **Ultrasound Examinations**: Regular ultrasound scans to assess fetal growth, amniotic fluid levels, and placental function.

4. **Education and Counseling**:
   - ➢ **Risk Awareness**: Educating parents about potential complications and signs of preterm labor or pregnancy-induced hypertension.

   - ➢ **Birth Planning**: Discussing birth options and preferences, including the possibility of cesarean delivery if indicated.

Preparing for Potential Complications

Anticipating and preparing for potential complications during a high-risk pregnancy can help ensure timely intervention and management.

1. **Gestational Diabetes**:
   - **Screening**: Testing for gestational diabetes around 24-28 weeks of pregnancy.

   - **Management**: Dietary modifications, blood glucose monitoring, and possibly insulin therapy under medical supervision.

2. **Hypertensive Disorders**:
   - **Preeclampsia**: Monitoring blood pressure and urinary protein levels regularly.

   - **Management**: Medications to control blood pressure and prevent complications for both mother and baby.

3. **Preterm Labor**:

> **Signs and Symptoms**: Educating parents about signs of preterm labor, such as regular contractions, pelvic pressure, or vaginal bleeding.

> **Management**: Administering corticosteroids to enhance fetal lung maturity if preterm birth is anticipated.

4. **Placental Issues**:

> **Placenta Previa or Abruptio**: Monitoring for symptoms such as vaginal bleeding and abdominal pain.

> **Management**: Depending on severity, bed rest, hospitalization, or early delivery may be necessary.

5. **Fetal Growth Restriction**:

> **Ultrasound Monitoring**: Assessing fetal growth and well-being to detect signs of growth restriction early.

➢ **Management**: Close surveillance and sometimes early delivery if fetal growth is significantly compromised.

Navigating a high-risk pregnancy involves proactive management, specialized prenatal care, and careful preparation for potential complications. By identifying risk factors early, collaborating with healthcare providers, and staying informed, parents can optimize outcomes and ensure the best possible care for both mother and baby.

CHAPTER TWELVE

MULTIPLE PREGNANCIES CARE

Multiple pregnancies, such as twins, triplets, or more, present unique challenges and require specialized care to ensure the health and well-being of both the mother and the babies. This chapter explores the distinctive challenges of carrying multiples, delivery options and associated risks, and the specific considerations for postpartum care.

UNIQUE CHALLENGES OF CARRYING MULTIPLES

Carrying multiple babies simultaneously introduces several challenges that differ from singleton pregnancies:

1. Increased Risk of Complications:

> **Preterm Birth**: Multiple pregnancies often result in preterm labor, with the risk increasing with the number of babies.

➢ **Gestational Diabetes and Hypertension**: Higher incidence due to increased demands on the mother's body.

➢ **Placental Issues**: Higher likelihood of placental abruption, placenta previa, or inadequate blood supply to one or more babies.

2. Physical Discomfort:

➢ **Weight Gain**: Rapid and significant weight gain places extra strain on the mother's body and joints.

➢ **Stretching of Uterus**:Uterine expansion to accommodate multiple babies can cause discomfort, back pain, and difficulty breathing.

3. Emotional and Psychological Impact:

➢ **Anxiety and Stress**: Concerns about pregnancy complications, premature birth, and managing care for multiple infants.

> **Logistical Challenges**: Planning for multiple births, including nursery preparation, childcare, and financial considerations.

4. **Nutritional Demands**:

> **Increased Nutrient Requirements**: Higher intake of calories, protein, vitamins, and minerals to support fetal growth and development.

> **Monitoring**: Close monitoring of maternal nutrition and weight gain to ensure adequate support for multiple babies.

Delivery Options and Risks

The method of delivery for multiples depends on various factors, including gestational age, fetal positions, and maternal health considerations:

1. **Vaginal Delivery**:

> - **Suitability**: Possible for twins and sometimes triplets if the first baby is in a head-down position (vertex).

> - **Careful Monitoring**: Continuous fetal monitoring during labor to detect any signs of distress.

2. **Cesarean Section** (C-Section):

> - **Indications**: Often recommended for higher-order multiples (triplets or more), breech presentations, or other complications.

> - **Timing**: Scheduled C-sections may be planned to minimize risks associated with labor and delivery.

3. **Risk of Preterm Birth**:

> - **Early Delivery**: Multiples are more likely to be born prematurely, requiring neonatal intensive care and specialized medical support.

> **Preparation**: Antenatal corticosteroids may be administered to enhance lung development in premature babies.

4. **Perinatal Risks**:

> **Complications**: Higher risk of low birth weight, developmental delays, and long-term health issues for multiples born prematurely.

> **Neonatal Care**: Immediate access to neonatal specialists and facilities equipped to handle multiple births.

POSTPARTUM CARE FOR MULTIPLES

Postpartum care for mothers of multiples focuses on recovery, breastfeeding support, and managing the needs of multiple infants:

1. **Physical Recovery**:

> **Monitoring**: Close observation for postpartum bleeding, infection, and healing of C-section incisions if applicable.

> **Pain Management**: Medications and strategies to alleviate discomfort and promote healing.

2. **Breastfeeding and Feeding Challenges**:

> **Establishing Feeding Routines**: Support for breastfeeding multiples, including positioning techniques and lactation consultation.

> **Supplemental Feeding**: Combination feeding with breast milk and formula may be necessary to meet the nutritional needs of all babies.

3. **Emotional Support**:

> **Postpartum Adjustment**: Coping with the demands of caring for multiple infants,

sleep deprivation, and emotional highs and lows.

> **Peer Support**: Connecting with other parents of multiples through support groups or online communities.

4. **Practical Considerations**:

> **Logistics**: Organizing caregiving responsibilities, scheduling feedings, and managing household tasks with support from family and friends.

> **Professional Assistance**: Hiring help, such as a doula or postpartum nurse, to assist with newborn care and household chores.

Managing a multiple pregnancy involves navigating unique challenges, making informed decisions about delivery options, and preparing for specialized postpartum care. By understanding these aspects and receiving comprehensive support from healthcare providers and loved ones, parents can optimize outcomes and ensure a positive experience welcoming their multiples into the world.

PART 5: RESOURCES AND SUPPORT

CHAPTER THIRTEEN

ADOPTION AND SURROGACY

Adoption and surrogacy are two distinct paths to parenthood that involve unique processes, emotional journeys, and considerations for postpartum care for adoptive and surrogate parents.

THE PROCESS AND EMOTIONAL JOURNEY

ADOPTION:

1. Initial Steps:

> **Decision to Adopt**: The choice to adopt, which can be motivated by a number of things including infertility, the need to grow a family, or a calling to give a needy kid a loving home, is the first step in the path.

➢ **Research and Education**: Prospective adoptive parents research adoption agencies, legal requirements, and types of adoption (domestic, international, foster care).

2. Home Study and Preparation:

➢ **Home Study**: Required by adoption agencies to assess the prospective parents' readiness, suitability, and home environment for raising a child.

➢ **Training and Education**: Adoption agencies often provide training on parenting skills, understanding adoption dynamics, and supporting the adopted child's emotional needs.

3. Matching and Placement:

➢ **Waiting Period**: Potential adoptive parents may wait for a match with a birth mother or child.

➢ **Legal Processes**: Finalizing the adoption through legal procedures, including consent, termination of parental rights, and adoption hearings.

4. **Emotional Challenges**:
> - **Expectation and Uncertainty**: Managing expectations and coping with uncertainties during the adoption process, including potential setbacks or changes in plans.
>
> - **Attachment and Bonding**: Building a bond with the adopted child, navigating attachment dynamics, and supporting the child's adjustment to a new family environment.

SURROGACY:

1. **Choosing Surrogacy**:

> - **Reasons for Surrogacy**: Surrogacy is chosen due to medical reasons, fertility challenges, or personal circumstances where carrying a pregnancy is not possible.
>
> - **Types of Surrogacy**: Traditional surrogacy (surrogate uses her own egg) vs.

gestational surrogacy (surrogate carries an embryo created from intended parents' or donor gametes).

2. **Legal and Medical Processes**:

➤ **Legal Agreements**: Drafting and signing legal contracts outlining rights, responsibilities, and financial agreements between the surrogate and intended parents.

➤ **Medical Procedures**: In vitro fertilization (IVF) process, embryo transfer, and prenatal care managed by reproductive specialists.

3. **Relationship Dynamics**:

➤ **Surrogate-Intended Parent Relationship**: Building a trusting relationship between the surrogate and intended parents, navigating communication, and respecting boundaries.

➤ **Supporting the Surrogate**: Providing emotional support and recognizing the surrogate's role in the journey to parenthood.

4. **Emotional Rollercoaster**:

- ➤ **Hope and Anxiety**: Balancing hope for a successful pregnancy with anxiety about potential complications or emotional challenges.

- ➤ **Joy of Parenthood**: Celebrating the birth of a child and adjusting to life as parents after the surrogacy journey.

POSTPARTUM CARE FOR ADOPTIVE AND SURROGATE PARENTS

ADOPTIVE PARENTS:

1. Transition to Parenthood:

- ➤ **Bonding and Attachment**: Building a strong bond with the adopted child through nurturing, caregiving, and creating a secure attachment.

- ➤ **Supporting the Child**: Addressing the child's emotional needs, helping them adjust to a new environment, and promoting a sense of belonging within the family.

2. Legal and Administrative Tasks:

- ➤ **Finalizing Adoption**: Completing legal procedures to finalize the adoption, including court hearings, parental rights, and obtaining a new birth certificate.

- ➤

> **Parental Responsibilities**: Assuming legal responsibilities for the child's well-being, education, healthcare, and financial support.

3. Emotional Well-Being:

> **Processing Emotions**: Managing feelings of joy, gratitude, anxiety, and adjustment challenges associated with becoming a parent through adoption.

> **Support Networks**: Seeking support from family, friends, and adoption support groups to share experiences, advice, and emotional support.

SURROGATE PARENTS:

1. Physical Recovery:

> **Postpartum Healing**: Supporting the surrogate's physical recovery after childbirth, including monitoring health, managing discomfort, and promoting rest.

➤ **Medical Check-ups**: Follow-up appointments with healthcare providers to ensure recovery and address any postpartum concerns.

2. Emotional Adjustment:

➤ **Transitioning Roles**: Navigating the emotional transition from pregnancy to post-surrogacy life, including feelings of fulfillment, separation, or loss.

➤ **Communication and Closure**: Maintaining open communication with intended parents about emotional experiences, expectations, and post-surrogacy relationships.

3. Support Systems:

➤ **Surrogate Community**: Connecting with other surrogates through support groups or online forums to share experiences, advice, and emotional support.

➤ **Professional Counseling**: Accessing counseling services to process emotions, address any psychological challenges, and prepare for life after surrogacy.

NOTE: Adoption and surrogacy journeys involve intricate processes, emotional highs and lows, and unique postpartum care considerations. By understanding these aspects and receiving comprehensive support from healthcare providers, adoption agencies, and support networks, parents can navigate these paths to parenthood with resilience and fulfillment.

CHAPTER FOURTEEN

BUILDING A SUPPORT NETWORK

Building a support network is crucial for navigating the challenges and joys of parenthood. This chapter explores the importance of family and friends, joining support groups, and utilizing community resources to create a robust support system.

IMPORTANCE OF FAMILY AND FRIENDS

1. Emotional Support:

> **Understanding and Empathy**: Family and friends offer emotional support by listening, providing encouragement, and empathizing with the ups and downs of parenthood.

> **Sharing Experiences**: Sharing personal experiences and advice can help new parents feel less isolated and more confident in their parenting journey.

2. **Practical Support:**

> **Assistance with Childcare**: Family and friends can help with childcare, allowing parents to take breaks and attend to personal needs.

> **Household Help**: Support with household chores, meal preparation, and errands lightens the load for new parents adjusting to their new routines.

3. **Bonding Opportunities:**

> **Building Relationships**: Grandparents, aunts, uncles, and close friends contribute to the child's extended support network, fostering strong family bonds.

> **Creating Memories**: Sharing special moments and milestones with loved ones enriches family experiences and creates lasting memories.

FINDING AND JOINING SUPPORT GROUPS

1. Types of Support Groups:

> **Parenting Groups**: Local parenting groups or online forums provide a platform for parents to connect, share tips, and seek advice on various parenting topics.

> **Specific Needs Groups**: Groups focused on topics such as breastfeeding, postpartum depression, single parenting, or special needs children offer targeted support.

2. Benefits of Support Groups:

> **Shared Experiences**: Connecting with other parents facing similar challenges validates experiences and reduces feelings of isolation.

> **Expert Advice**: Access to expert advice from healthcare professionals, lactation consultants, and experienced parents within the group.

3. Online and In-Person Groups:

> **Convenience**: Online groups offer flexibility for busy parents to participate from home, while in-person groups provide opportunities for face-to-face interaction and networking.

>

> **Social Support**: Building friendships and networks of support that extend beyond parenting topics, fostering a sense of community and belonging.

UTILIZING COMMUNITY RESOURCES

1. **Parenting Classes and Workshops**:

> **Education and Skill-Building**: Community centers, hospitals, and local organizations offer classes on newborn care,

breastfeeding, infant CPR, and parenting techniques.

> **Networking Opportunities**: Attendees can connect with other parents, share insights, and build supportive relationships.

2. **Childcare and Parenting Services**:

> **Daycare Centers**: Researching and selecting reputable daycare centers or childcare providers that align with parenting values and preferences.

> **Parenting Hotlines**: Accessing helplines or resources for immediate support and guidance on parenting issues or concerns.

3. **Healthcare and Mental Health Services**:

> **Pediatricians and Family Doctors**: Choosing healthcare providers who prioritize parental involvement, provide reliable medical advice, and support child development.

➢ **Help for Mental Health**: identifying the symptoms of postpartum depression or anxiety and getting professional assistance from mental health professionals such as therapists, counselors, or support groups.

Building a support network is essential for parents to navigate the challenges of parenthood effectively. By leveraging the support of family and friends, joining relevant support groups, and utilizing community resources, parents can access emotional support, practical assistance, and valuable knowledge to enhance their parenting journey.

CHAPTER FIFTEEN

PROFESSIONAL HELP

Professional help plays a crucial role in supporting parents through the challenges and transitions of parenthood. This chapter focuses on choosing healthcare providers, recognizing when to seek professional mental health support, and understanding the roles of lactation consultants and postpartum doulas.

CHOOSING HEALTHCARE PROVIDERS

1. **Obstetrician/Gynecologist (OB/GYN):**

> **Role**: Provides prenatal care, monitors fetal development, and manages the health of the mother during pregnancy.

- ➢ **Choosing Criteria**: Consider qualifications, experience with high-risk pregnancies if applicable, communication style, and hospital affiliations.

2. **Pediatrician**:

- ➢ **Role**:Specializes in the health and development of infants, children, and adolescents.

- ➢ **Choosing Criteria**: Look for a pediatrician who shares your parenting philosophy, is accessible for appointments and emergencies, and provides comprehensive care.

3. **Family Doctor**:

- ➢ **Role**: Offers primary care services for the entire family, including prenatal care, pediatric care, and ongoing healthcare needs.

- ➢ **Choosing Criteria**: Evaluate their experience with newborns, accessibility, and ability to coordinate care across family members.

4. **Specialists**:

> **Lactation Consultant**: Provides expert guidance and support for breastfeeding challenges, including latching difficulties, low milk supply, and pumping advice.

> **Postpartum Doula**: Offers practical support, emotional encouragement, and education to new parents during the postpartum period, focusing on maternal recovery and newborn care.

When to Get Help for Mental Health Professionals

1. **Postpartum Depression and Anxiety**:

> **Symptoms**: Persistent sadness, anxiety, mood swings, difficulty bonding with the baby, and changes in appetite or sleep patterns.

> **Seeking Help**: Consult with a therapist, counselor, or psychiatrist if symptoms

persist for more than two weeks or interfere with daily functioning.

2. **Adjustment Challenges**:

> **Transition to Parenthood**: Feelings of overwhelm, stress, or difficulty adjusting to new roles and responsibilities.

> **Therapeutic Support**: Counseling or support groups can provide strategies for coping with changes and enhancing family dynamics.

3. **Trauma or Loss**:

> **Birth Complications**: Processing emotions related to birth trauma, unexpected outcomes, or loss during pregnancy or childbirth.

> **Therapeutic Interventions**: Trauma-informed care and specialized support can aid in healing and resilience.

Lactation Consultants and Postpartum Doulas

1. **Lactation Consultants**:

> **Role**: Assess breastfeeding challenges, provide education on proper latch techniques, positioning, and troubleshooting milk supply issues.

> **Benefits**: Support for establishing a successful breastfeeding relationship, addressing concerns promptly, and promoting maternal-infant bonding.

2. **Postpartum Doulas**:

> **Role**: Offer practical assistance with newborn care, including feeding, soothing techniques, light household chores, and emotional support for parents.

> **Benefits**: Reduce parental stress, enhance recovery for mothers, and facilitate a smoother transition into parenthood through knowledgeable guidance and compassionate care.

3. **Working Together**:

> **Collaborative Approach**: Lactation consultants and postpartum doulas work collaboratively with healthcare providers to ensure holistic support for families.

> **Continued Support**: Availability for ongoing consultations, follow-up visits, and resources to address evolving needs and challenges.

Accessing professional help enhances parental confidence, promotes optimal health outcomes for both parents and infants, and fosters a supportive environment during the early stages of parenthood. Carefully selecting healthcare professionals, knowing when to seek mental health help, and using the skills of lactation consultants and postpartum doulas are ways that parents may manage the challenges and rewards of parenting with compassionate care and knowledgeable direction.

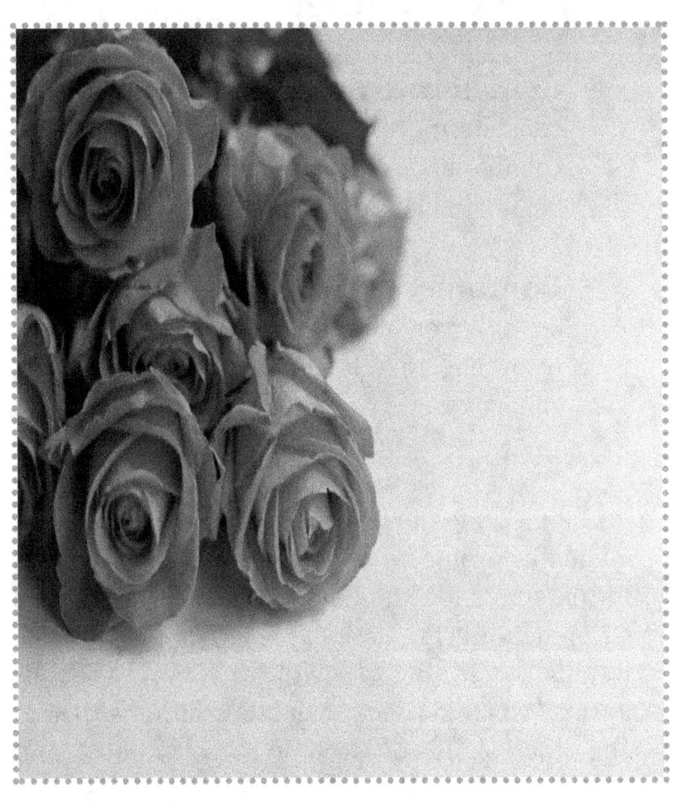

CHAPTER SIXTEEN

REFLECTING ON THE JOURNEY

Reflecting on the journey of parenthood involves embracing the changes and challenges, celebrating milestones and growth, and looking forward to the future with optimism and resilience.

Embracing the Changes and Challenges

Parenthood brings about profound changes and challenges, each offering opportunities for personal growth and learning:

1. **Adjusting to Parenthood**:

> - **Shift in Priorities**: Embracing the transformation from individual-focused to family-centered priorities, including sleep schedules, daily routines, and career adjustments.

> - **Adapting Roles**: Navigating new roles as caregivers, partners, and role models for children, fostering resilience and flexibility in the face of evolving responsibilities.

2. **Navigating Challenges**:

> - **Parenting Styles**: Finding a balance between nurturing and setting boundaries, adjusting to each child's unique needs and personalities.

> - **Communication**: Enhancing communication skills within the family unit, fostering trust, and promoting open dialogue to address challenges effectively.

3. **Coping with Setbacks**:

> - **Resilience**: Building resilience to manage unexpected challenges, setbacks, or

parenting difficulties, seeking support from loved ones, professionals, or community resources.

> **Self-Care**: Prioritizing self-care practices to maintain physical health, emotional well-being, and sustainable energy levels throughout parenthood.

Celebrating Milestones and Growth

Parenting is a journey marked by significant milestones and personal growth for both parents and children:

1. **Child Development**: Celebrating developmental milestones such as first steps, first words, and academic achievements, recognizing the growth and potential of each child.

> **Parental Pride**: Expressing pride and joy in witnessing children's accomplishments, fostering a supportive environment for exploration and learning.

2. **Family Bonding**: Creating meaningful traditions, routines, and shared experiences that strengthen family bonds and create lasting memories.

> **Quality Time**: Prioritizing quality time together through activities, outings, and shared interests that nurture connection and mutual understanding.

3. **Parental Growth**: Reflecting on personal growth as individuals and as parents, learning from experiences, and adapting parenting strategies based on insights and feedback.

> **Learning Curve**: Embracing the learning curve of parenthood, acknowledging mistakes as opportunities for growth, and seeking continuous improvement in parenting practices.

LOOKING FORWARD TO THE FUTURE

As parents reflect on their journey, they also envision a future filled with hope, dreams, and possibilities:

1. **Setting Goals**: Establishing short-term and long-term goals for family well-being, educational aspirations for children, and personal achievements

   ➢ **Vision for Children**: Nurturing children's interests, talents, and aspirations, supporting them in exploring opportunities and pursuing their passions.

2. **Family Planning**: Considering future family planning decisions, including sibling dynamics, career aspirations, and financial goals.

   ➢ **Support Systems**: Cultivating a supportive network of family, friends, and community resources to provide guidance, encouragement, and assistance along the way.

3. **Legacy of Parenthood**: Reflecting on the legacy of parenthood, including values passed down to children, memories shared, and the impact of parental love and support on future generations.

> **Optimism**: Embracing optimism and resilience in facing challenges, fostering a positive outlook on the journey ahead, and cherishing the bonds that define the family's journey through parenthood.

Reflecting on the journey of parenthood encompasses embracing transformation, celebrating achievements, and envisioning a future filled with hope and opportunities. By navigating changes with resilience, celebrating milestones with pride, and looking forward with optimism, parents can cultivate a fulfilling and meaningful journey through the joys and challenges of raising children.

CONCLUSION

Congratulations on completing the journey through "Pregnancy and Postpartum Care." With in-depth analyses and helpful guidance to accompany you at every turn, this ebook has walked you through the life-changing experiences of pregnancy, childbirth, and the early years of parenthood.

Reflecting on Your Journey

As you reflect on the chapters within this book, remember the milestones you've achieved and the challenges you've overcome. From the excitement of discovering pregnancy to the anticipation and preparation for labor, each phase has been a testament to your strength and resilience. Through understanding pregnancy stages, managing symptoms, preparing for childbirth, and embracing the postpartum period, you've navigated with knowledge and confidence.

Embracing Parenthood

Parenthood is a continuous journey of learning and growth, marked by moments of joy, discovery, and occasional uncertainty. Embrace the changes in your life, both as an individual and as a family unit. Recognize the importance of self-care, nurturing relationships, and seeking support from healthcare providers, family, and friends. Remember that it's okay to seek help when needed and to trust your instincts as a parent.

Looking Ahead

As you look towards the future, envision the dreams and aspirations you hold for yourself and your growing family. Whether you're welcoming your first child or expanding your family, your journey is unique and filled with promise. Continue to prioritize your well-being, nurture your relationships, and foster a supportive environment for your children to thrive.

Gratitude

Lastly, I extend my heartfelt gratitude for allowing me to be a part of your journey through this ebook. It's been an honor to share knowledge and insights that I hope have empowered and enriched your experience of pregnancy and early parenthood. Remember, every experience, challenge, and moment of joy contributes to the beautiful tapestry of parenthood.

Wishing you and your family health, happiness, and cherished memories as you embark on this remarkable journey of parenthood.

With warm regards,

Danielle Wallace

www.ingramcontent.com/pod-product-compliance
Lightning Source LLC
Chambersburg PA
CBHW061642250726